The Easy Lean Breakfast C

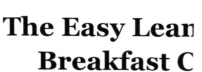

50 easy-to-prepare and delicious recipes for your lean and green breakfast, to start the day and boost energy

Josephine Reed

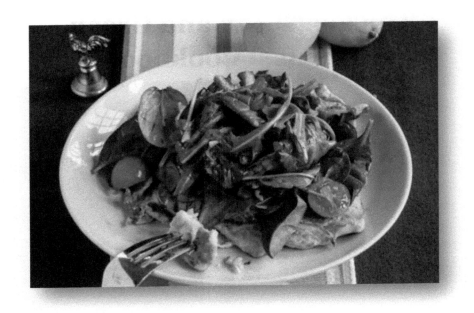

Please consult a licensed professional before attempting any techniques outlined in this book.

By reading this document, the reader agrees that under no circumstances is the author responsible for any losses, direct or indirect, which are incurred as a result of the use of information contained within this document, including, but not limited to, — errors, omissions, or inaccuracies.

Table of contents

Quinoa Porridge

Prep Time: 5 minutes

Cook Time: 25 minutes

Serve: 2

Ingredients:

- 2 cups of coconut milk
- 1 cup rinsed quinoa
- 1/8 tsp. ground cinnamon
- 1 cup fresh blueberries

Instructions:

1. In a saucepan, boil the coconut milk over high heat.

2. Add the quinoa to the milk, then bring the mixture to a boil.

3. You then let it simmer for 15 minutes on medium heat until the milk is reduced.

4. Add the cinnamon, then mix it properly in the saucepan.

5. Cover the saucepan and cook for at least 8 minutes until the milk is completely absorbed.

6. Add in the blueberries, then cook for 30 more seconds.

Nutrition: Calories: 271 kcal Fat: 3.7g Carbs: 54g Protein:6.5g

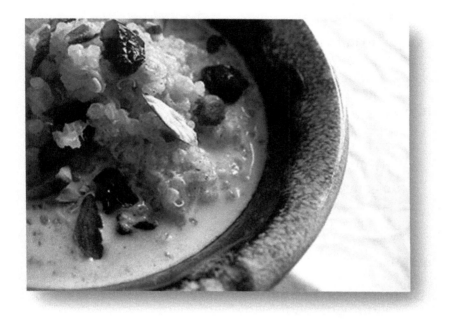

Amaranth Porridge

Prep Time: 5 minutes

Cook Time: 30 minutes

Serve: 2.

Ingredients:

- 2 cups of coconut milk
- 2 cups alkaline water
- 1 cup amaranth
- 2 tbsps. coconut oil
- 1 tbsp. ground cinnamon

Instructions:

1. In a saucepan, mix the milk with water, then boil the mixture.

2. You stir in the amaranth, then reduce the heat to medium.

3. Cook on medium heat and then simmer for at least 30 minutes as you occasionally stir it.

4. Turn off the heat.

5. Add in cinnamon and coconut oil, then stir.

Nutrition: Calories: 434 kcal Fat: 35g Carbs: 27g Protein: 6.7g

Banana Barley Porridge

Prep Time: 15 minutes

Cook Time: 5 minutes

Serve: 2

Ingredients:

- 1 cup divided unsweetened coconut milk 1 small peeled and sliced banana 1/2 cup barley
- 3 drops liquid stevia
- 1/4 cup chopped coconuts

Instructions:

1. In a bowl, properly mix barley with half of the coconut milk and stevia.

2. Cover the mixing bowl, then refrigerate for about 6 hours.

3. In a saucepan, mix the barley mixture with coconut milk.

4. Cook for about 5 minutes on moderate heat.

5. Then top it with the chopped coconuts and the banana slices.

Nutrition: Calories: 159kcal Fat: 8.4g Carbs: 19.8g Proteins: 4.6g

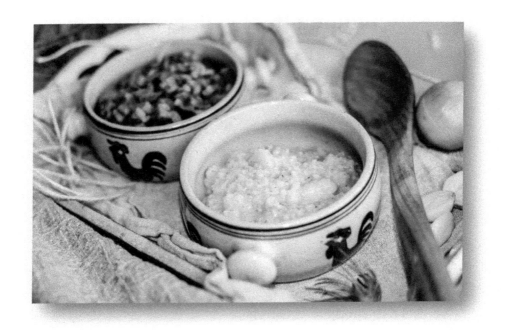

Zucchini Muffins

Prep Time: 10 minutes

Cook Time: 25 minutes

Serve: 16

Ingredients:

- 1 tbsp. ground flaxseed
- 3 tbsps. alkaline water
- 1/4 cup walnut butter
- 3 medium over-ripe bananas
- 2 small grated
- zucchinis
- 1/2 cup coconut milk
- 1 tsp. vanilla extract
- 2 cups coconut flour
- 1 tbsp. baking powder
- 1 tsp. cinnamon
- 1/4 tsp. sea salt

Instructions:

1. Tune the temperature of your oven to 375ºF.

2. Grease the muffin tray with the cooking spray.

3. In a bowl, mix the flaxseed with water.

4. In a glass bowl, mash the bananas, then stir in the remaining ingredients.

5. Properly mix and then divide the mixture into the muffin tray.

6. Bake it for 25 minutes.

Nutrition: Calories: 127 kcal Fat: 6.6g Carbs: 13g Protein: 0.7g

Millet Porridge

Prep Time: 10 minutes

Cook Time: 20 minutes

Serve: 2

Ingredients:

- Sea salt
- 1 tbsp. finely chopped coconuts
- 1/2 cup unsweetened coconut milk
- 1/2 cup rinsed and drained millet
- 1-1/2 cups alkaline water
- 3 drops liquid stevia

Instructions:

1. Sauté the millet in a non-stick skillet for about 3 minutes.

2. Add salt and water, then stir.

3. Let the meal boil, then reduce the amount of heat.

4. Cook for 15 minutes, then add the remaining ingredients. Stir.

5. Cook the meal for 4 extra minutes.

6. Serve the meal with toping of the chopped nuts.

Nutrition: Calories: 219 kcal Fat: 4.5g Carbs: 38.2g Protein: 6.4g

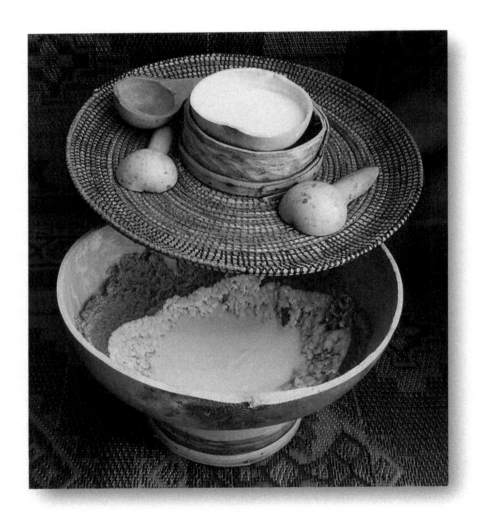

Jackfruit Vegetable Fry

Prep Time: 5 minutes

Cook Time: 5 minutes

Serve: 6

Ingredients:

- 2 finely chopped small onions
- 2 cups finely chopped cherry tomatoes
- 1/8 tsp. ground turmeric
- 1 tbsp. olive oil
- 2 seeded and chopped red bell peppers
- 3 cups seeded and chopped firm jackfruit
- 1/8 tsp. cayenne pepper
- 2 tbsps. chopped fresh basil leaves
- Salt

Instructions:

1. In a greased skillet, sauté the onions and bell peppers for about 5 minutes.

2. Add the tomatoes, then stir.

3. Cook for 2 minutes.

4. Then add the jackfruit, cayenne pepper, salt, and turmeric.

5. Cook for about 8 minutes.

6. Garnish the meal with basil leaves.

Nutrition: Calories: 236 kcal Fat: 1.8g Carbs: 48.3g Protein: 7g

Zucchini Pancakes with Jalapeno peppers

Prep Time: 15 minutes

Cook Time: 8 minutes

Serve: 8

Ingredients:

- 12 tbsps. alkaline water
- 6 large grated zucchinis
- Sea salt
- 4 tbsps. ground Flax Seeds
- 2 tips. olive oil
- 2 finely chopped jalapeño peppers
- 1/2 cup finely chopped scallions

Instructions:

1. In a bowl, mix water and the flax seeds, then set it aside.

2. Pour oil into a large non-stick skillet, then heat it on medium heat.

3. The add the black pepper, salt, and zucchini.

4. Cook for 3 minutes, then transfer the zucchini into a large bowl.

5. Add the flaxseed and the scallion mixture, then properly mix it.

6. Preheat a griddle, then grease it lightly with the cooking spray.

7. Pour 1/4 of the zucchini mixture into the griddle, then cook for 3 minutes.

8. Flip the side carefully, then cook for 2 more minutes.

9. Repeat the procedure with the remaining mixture in batches.

Nutrition: Calories: 71 kcal Fat: 2.8g Carbs: 9.8g Protein: 3.7g

Squash Hash

Prep Time: 2 minutes

Cook Time: 10 minutes

Serve: 2

Ingredients:

- 1 tsp. onion powder
- 1/2 cup finely chopped onion
- 2 cups spaghetti squash
- 1/2 tsp. sea salt

Instructions:

1. Using paper towels, squeeze extra moisture from spaghetti squash.

2. Place the squash into a bowl, then add the salt, onion, and onion powder.

3. Stir properly to mix them.

4. Spray a non-stick cooking skillet with cooking spray, then place it over moderate heat.

5. Add the spaghetti squash to the pan.

6. Cook the squash for about 5 minutes.

7. Flip the hash browns using a spatula.

8. Cook for 5 minutes until the desired crispness is reached.

Nutrition: Calories: 44 kcal Fat: 0.6g Carbs: 9.7g Protein: 0.9

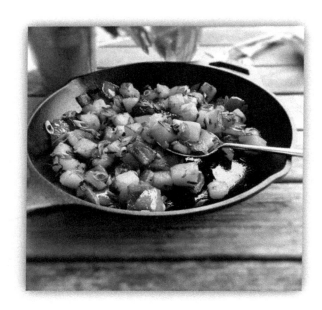

Hemp Seed Porridge

Prep Time: 5 minutes

Cook Time: 5 minutes

Serve: 6

Ingredients:

- 3 cups cooked hemp seed
- 1 packet Stevia
- 1 cup of coconut milk

Instructions:

1. In a saucepan, mix the rice and the coconut milk over moderate heat for about 5 minutes as you stir it constantly.

2. Take the pan out of the burner, then add it to the Stevia. Stir.

3. Serve in 6 bowls.

Nutrition: Calories: 236 kcal Fat: 1.8g Carbs: 48.3g Protein: 7g

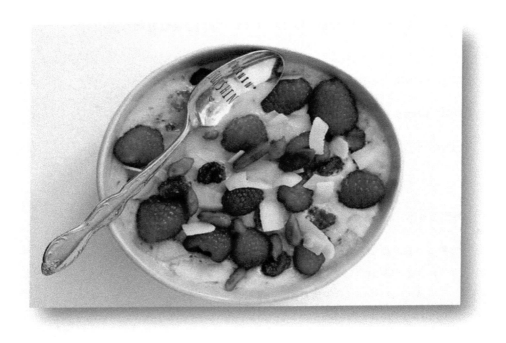

Pumpkin Spice Quinoa

Prep Time: 10 minutes

Cook Time: 0 minutes

Serve: 2

Ingredients:

- 1 cup cooked quinoa
- 1 cup unsweetened coconut milk
- 1 large mashed banana
- 1/4 cup pumpkin puree
- 1 tsp. pumpkin spice
- 2 tips. chia seeds

Instructions:

1. In a container, mix all the ingredients.

2. Seal the lid, then shake the container properly to mix.

3. Refrigerate overnight.

Nutrition: Calories: 212 kcal Fat: 11.9g Carbs: 31.7g Protein: 7.3g

Healthy Greek Salmon Salad

Prep Time: 10 minutes

Cook Time: 8 minutes

Serve: 4

Ingredients:

- ¼ cup olive oil
- 3 tablespoons red wine vinegar
- 2 tablespoons freshly crush lemon juice (from 1 lemon)
- 1 clove of garlic, chopped
- ¾ teaspoon dried oregano
- 1/2 teaspoon Kosar salt
- ¼ teaspoon fresh black pepper
- One finely chopped red onion
- A cup of cold water
- 4 (6 oz) salmon fillets, peeled
- 2 medium-sized Korean salads, such as Boston or Bibb (about 1 kilogram), broken into bite-size pieces
- 2 medium-sized tomatoes, cut into 1-inch pieces
- 1 medium English cucumber, quadrilateral and then cut into 1/2-inch pieces
- ½ cup of half-length Kalamata olives 4 oz Feta Cheese, minced (about 1 cup)

Instructions:

1. In the middle of the oven, arrange a shelf and heat to 425 degrees Fahrenheit. While the oven is warming, marinate the salmon and soften the onion (instructions below).

2. Put the olive oil, vinegar, lemon juice, garlic, oregano, salt and pepper in a large bowl, then transfer three tablespoons of vinegar large enough into a baking dish to keep all the salmon chunks in one layer. Add the salmon, lightly rotate a few times to wrap evenly in the wings. Cover the fridge. Pour the onion and water into a small bowl and set aside 10 minutes to make the onion stronger. Drain and release the liquid.

3. Discover the salmon and grill for 8 to 12 minutes until they are cooked and lightly fried. Thermometer instant-read in the middle of the thickest tab should record 120 degrees Fahrenheit to 130 degrees Fahrenheit for the rare medium or 135 degrees Fahrenheit to 145 degrees Fahrenheit. The cooking depends on the thickness of the salmon, depending on the thickest portion of the fillet. It Al depends on the salad.

4. Add the salad, tomatoes, cucumbers, olives, and red onion to the Gina Vine bowl and salt to combine. Divide into four plates or shallow bowl. When the salmon is ready, place one fillet over each salad. Sprinkle with feta and serve quickly.

Nutrition: Calories: 351 Total fat: 4g Cholesterol: 94mg Fiber: 2g Protein: 12g Sodium: 327mg

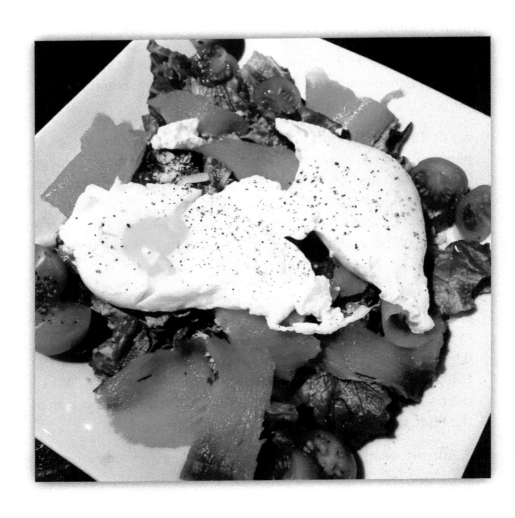

Mediterranean Pepper

Prep Time: 5 minutes

Cook Time: 20 minutes

Serve: 4

Ingredients:

- 1/2 teaspoon restrained oil 1/2 cup sun-dried tomatoes
- 2 cups of spinach (fresh or frozen)
- 1/2 spoon drops of zaatar spices
- 10 eggs, screaming
- 1/2 cup Feta cheese
- 1-2 tablespoons
- salt and pepper

Instructions:

1. At 350 degrees Fahrenheit, firstly preheat the oven

2. Heat a cast-iron boiler over medium heat. Add the olive oil and peas, slowly and slowly cooking until you want to release the liquid and start to brown and brown. Then, sauté the sun-dried tomatoes with a little reserved oil, spinach and zucchini, and cook for 2-3 minutes until the spinach is crushed.

3. When the spinach has faded, pour the vegetable mixture evenly into the cast iron fish and then add the boiled eggs, turning the pan so that the eggs cover the vegetables evenly. Bake on medium heat

until the eggs start about halfway through. Pour the eggs and vegetables with the spatula into the pan, leave the eggs to cook until the frittata is placed.

4. When the eggs are almost half cooked, add the Feta cheese and spoon the horseradish sauce on top and dust with salt and pepper. Remove the cast iron from the oven and place it in the middle rack in the oven. Bake until cooked on the ferrite; it will take about five minutes.

5. Bring out from the oven and let it cool slightly. For cedar, cut or square the pie and pour with a pan.

Nutrition: Calories: 311 Total fat: 4g Cholesterol: 84mg Fiber: 2g Protein: 12g Sodium: 357mg

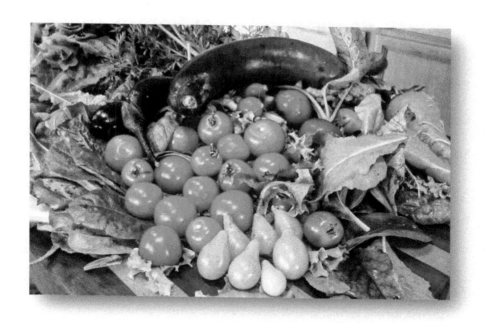

Black Beans and Sweet Potato Tacos

Prep Time: 10 minutes

Cook Time: 30 minutes

Serve: 6

Ingredients:

- 1 lb. sweet potato (about 2 medium teaspoons), skin cut and cut
- into 1/2-inch pieces
- Divide into 2 tablespoons of olive oil
- 1 tablespoon Kosar salt, divided
- ¼ teaspoon fresh black pepper on large white or yellow onion, finely chopped
- 2 teaspoons of red pepper
- 1 cumin with a teaspoon
- 1 (15 oz.) can be black beans, drained and drained Cup of water
- ¼ cup freshly chopped garlic
- 12 pcs. Corn
- To serving guacamole
- Sliced cheese or feta cheese (optional)
- Wood Wedge

Instructions:

1. In the oven, set out a shelf in the middle and place to 425 degrees Fahrenheit. Set a big sheet of aluminum foil on the work surface. Collect the tortillas from the top and wrap them completely in foil. Put it aside

2. Put sweet potatoes on a small baking sheet. Mix with one tablespoon oil and sprinkle with 1/2 teaspoon salt and 1/4 teaspoon black pepper. Discard to mix and play in one layer. Fry for 20 minutes. Sprinkle the potatoes with a flat lid and set aside until a corner of the oven is clear.

3. Put the foil wrapping in the space and continue to cook for about 10 minutes until the sweet potatoes are browned and stained and the seasonings are heated. Also, cook the beans.

4. You then heat one tablespoon remaining in a large skillet over low heat. Put the onion and cook, occasionally stirring, until translucent, about 3 minutes. Mix the pepper powder, cumin, and 1/2 teaspoon salt. Add the beans and water.

5. Shield the pan and reduce the heat to low heat. Cook for 5 minutes, then slice and use the fork's back to chop the beans a little, about half of the total. If water still remains in the vessel, stir the exposed mixture for about 30 seconds until evaporated.

6. Peel the sweet potatoes and add the cantaloupe to the black beans, and mix. If used, fill the yolk with a mixture of black beans and top with guacamole and cheese. Serve with lime wedges.

Nutrition: Calories: 251 Total fat: 4g Cholesterol: 94mg Fiber: 2g Protein: 15g Sodium: 329mg

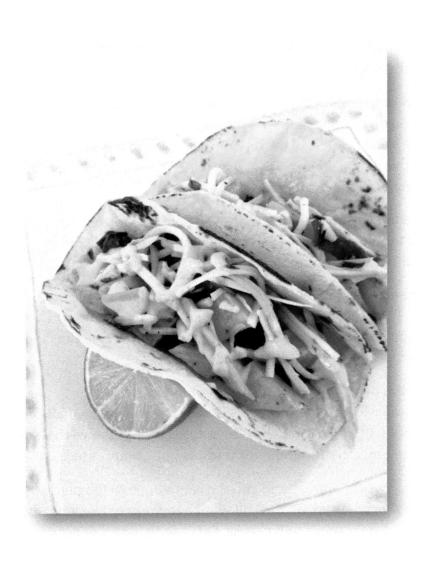

Seafood Cooked from Beer

Prep Time: 30 minutes

Cook Time: 1 hour

Serve: 8

Ingredients:

Seafood:

- Canola oil for roasting
- 1/2 Cup Coarse cornmeal
- 1/2 tablespoon red pepper
- 1/4 baking soda
- 1 1/2 Cup Flour for all purposes is divided
- Kosher salt and freshly ground black pepper
- 1 12 oz can drink beer in style
- 1 code and skin without skin, cut into 8 strips
- 1 large cup (number 25/25) of peeled and spread shrimp (remaining tail)
- 16 percentiles, shake
- 1 lemon sliced with cedar wedge
- Tartar sauce, mignon, chimichurri, hot sauce, and malt vinegar, for cedar.

Sos tartar:

- 1/2 Cup Mayonnaise
- 2 teaspoons, pickled, chopped or pureed
- 1 tablespoon fresh lemon juice

- 1 tablespoon three-quarter pants
- 1 tablespoon mustard
- Kosher salt and freshly ground black pepper
- 1/2 cup Red wine vinegar
- 1 small rest, finely chopped

Kosher salt and chimichurri of freshly ground black pepper:

- 1/2 Cup Fresh parsley on a flat-leaf
- 1/4 Cup White wine vinegar
- 2 tablespoons olive oil
- 2 cloves of minced garlic
- 1 stem, seeds and mincemeat
- 1 tablespoon fresh oregano, chopped
- Sare Kosar

Instructions:

1. Heat 1 1/2-inch oil in a large Dutch oven over medium heat at 375 degrees F (deep-fried temperature with a thermometer).

2. Meanwhile, chop corn, bell pepper, baking soda, 1 cup of flour, 1/2 teaspoon salt, and 1/2 teaspoon pepper in a bowl. Add the broth and the phloem to mix.

3. Put 1/2 cup of the remaining flour in a bowl. Add salt, pepper and the fish, shrimps, shells, and lemon slices, and serve little.

4. Work several pieces at once, remove the seafood and the lemons from the flour, shake too much, drain the dough and allow the excess drops to return to the container. Carefully add the hot oil, being careful not to overload the pot. Roast golden brown and

cook for 1 to 2 minutes. Transfer to a sheet of paper towel —
season with salt.

5. Make the tartar sauce: mayonnaise, pickled or mixed the cloves,
and pour the lemon juice, pepper, and mustard whole in a bowl.
Season with Kosar salt and freshly ground pepper; feel free to add
more lemon juice. Face 2/3 glass.

6. To Make a Mignonette: add red wine vinegar and finely minced
mustard in a bowl. Season with Kosar salt and freshly ground
pepper; allow standing for at least 30 minutes or up to 24 hours.
Make 1/2 cup.

7. Make Chimichurri: Combine parsley, white wine vinegar, olive
oil, garlic, jalapeño, and fresh oregano in a bowl. It is seasoned
with Kosar salt. Face 2/3 glass.

8. It is served with lemon wedges, tartar sauce, mignon, chemicals,
hot sauce, and malt vinegar.

Nutrition: Calories: 221 Total fat: 4g Cholesterol: 94mg Fiber: 2g
Protein: 12g Sodium: 327mg

Crab Chicken

Prep Time: 20 minutes

Cook Time: 40 minutes

Serve: 8

Ingredients:

- Canola oil for roasting
- 1c coarse cornflour
- 1/2 Cup Flour, spoon, and surface used
- 3/4 Cup Baking powder
- 1/2 spoon
- 1/4 tablespoon
- Sare Kosar
- 2 graphic, finely chopped
- 1 tablespoon crushed peas
- Eat 8 ounces of claw crab meat (2.11 c)
- 4 oz. of Gruyère cheese, chilled (about 1 cup)
- 1 c Dough water
- 1 you tie

Instructions:

1. Heat 1 1/2-inch oil in a large Dutch oven over medium heat up to 350 degrees F (deep-fry).

2. Meanwhile, mix the cornmeal, flour, baking powder, cayenne, baking soda, and 3/4 teaspoon salt in a bowl. Add onion and onion and mix to combine. Add the crab meat and cheese and mix with a fork to combine. In the center of a well, add the butter and egg and mix to combine.

3. Spoon soup into the hot oil and be careful not to spill the pan and fry, occasionally turning until browned, 3 to 5 minutes. Transfer toa sheet of paper towel — season with salt repeat with the remaining dough.

Nutrition: Calories: 351 Total fat: 4g Cholesterol: 94mg Fiber: 2g Protein: 12g Sodium: 319mg

Slow Lentil Soup

Prep Time: 10 minutes

Cook Time: 20 minutes

Serve: 6

Ingredients:

- 4 cups (1 quart) of low sodium vegetable juice
- 1 (14 oz.) tomatoes can (no leak)
- 1 small, fried yellow onion
- 1 medium carrot, sliced
- 1 medium-sized celery stalk, one-piece
- 1 cup green lentils
- 1 teaspoon of olive oil, plus more for cedar
- 2 cloves of garlic, turn
- 1 teaspoon Kosar salt
- 1 teaspoon tomato paste
- 1 leaf
- 1/2 teaspoon below ground
- 1/2 teaspoon of ground coriander
- 1/4 teaspoon of smoked peppers
- 2 tablespoons red wine vinegar
- Serving options: plain yogurt, olive oil, freshly chopped parsley or coriander leaves

Instructions:

1. Put all ingredients, except vinegar, in a slow cooker for 1/3 to 2-4 quarts and mix to combine. Cover and cook in the LOW settings for about 8 hours until the lentil is tender.

2. Remove bay leaf and mix in red wine vinegar. If desired, place a pot, a drop of olive oil and fresh parsley or crushed liquid in a bowl.

Nutrition: Calories: 231 Total fat: 4g Cholesterol: 64mg Fiber: 2g Protein: 12g Sodium: 368mg

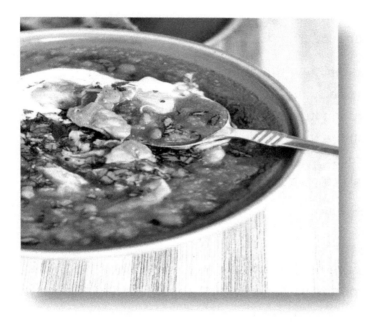

Light Bang Shrimp Paste

Prep Time: 10 minutes

Cook Time: 20 minutes

Serve: 4

Ingredients:

For crunchy crumbs:

- 1 tablespoon oil without butter
- Fresh cups or pancakes
- 1/8 teaspoon Kosar salt
- 1/8 teaspoon fresh black pepper
- Pepper racks
- Spend garlic powder

For shrimp pasta:

- Cooking spray
- ½ cup of Greek yogurt whole milk
- 2 tablespoons of Asian sweet pepper sauce, such as the iconic eel
- 1 teaspoon of honey
- ¼ teaspoon of garlic powder
- The juice is divided into 2 medium lemons (about 1/4 glass)
- 12 ounces of dried spaghetti
- 1 cup shrimp without skin and peeled
- 1 teaspoon Kosar salt, plus for pasta juice

- ¼ teaspoon fresh black pepper
- 1/8 teaspoon cayenne pepper
- 2 Moderated onions, sliced, sliced

Instructions:

1. Make crisp crumbs:

2. Over low heat, defrost the butter in a skillet. Add crumbs, salt, black pepper, cayenne pepper, and garlic powder. Cook while constantly stirring, until golden, crispy and fragrant. It will take 4 - 5 minutes, then put it aside.

3. Make shrimps:

4. Place a shelf in the middle of the oven and heat to 400 degrees

 Fahrenheit. Cover with a lightly cooked baking sheet with cooking spray. Put it aside

5. Boil salt water in a big pot. Meanwhile, chop yogurt, pepper sauce, honey, garlic powder and half of the lemon juice in a small bowl. Put it aside

6. Add the pasta when the water boils and boil the pasta for up to 10 minutes, or as directed. Dry the shrimps and place them on a sheet of ready-made cooking. Season with salt, black pepper and coffee and mix to cook. It stretches in a uniform layer. Roast once, until the shrimps are matte and pink, 6 to 8 minutes. Pour the remaining lemon juice over the shrimps, pour over it and pour the flavored pieces onto the baking sheet.

7. Evacuate the pasta and return it to the pot. Pour into the yogurt sauce and serve until well cooked. Put shrimp and juice on a

baking sheet with half of the onion and lightly add it again. Generously sprinkle each portion with a crunchy crumb and remaining onion. Serve immediately.

Nutrition: Calories: 351 Total fat: 4g Cholesterol: 94mg Fiber: 2g Protein: 12g Sodium: 327mg

Sweet and Smoked Salmon

Prep Time: 35 minutes

Cook Time: 1 hour

Serve: 8

Ingredients:

- 2 tablespoons light brown sugar
- 2 tablespoons smoked peppers
- 1 tablespoon shaved lemon peel
- Sare Kosar
- Freshly chopped black pepper
- Salmon fillets on the skin 1/2 kilogram

Instructions:

1. Soak a large plate (about 15 cm by 7 inches) in water for 1 to 2 hours.

2. It is heated over medium heat. Combine sugar, pepper, lemon zest, and 1/2 teaspoon of salt and pepper in a bowl. Mix the salmon with the salt and rub the mixture of spices in all parts of the meat.

3. Put the salmon on the wet plate, skin down — oven, covered, in the desired color, 25 to 28 minutes for medium.

Nutrition: Calories: 321 Total fat: 4g Cholesterol: 54mg Fiber: 2g
Protein: 12g Sodium: 337mg

Chocolate Cherry Crunch Granola

Prep Time: 10 minutes

Cook Time: 20 minutes

Serve: 6

Ingredients:

- 3 cups rolled oats
- 2 cups assorted seeds, such as sesame, chia, sunflower, and pepitas (hulled pumpkin seeds)
- 1 cup sliced almonds
- 1 cup unsweetened coconut flakes
- 2 teaspoons vanilla extract
- 2 teaspoons ground cinnamon
- 1 teaspoon fine sea salt
- ½ cup of cocoa powder
- ½ cup pure maple syrup
- ¼ cup coconut oil or canola oil
- 1 cup dried cherries (unsweetened, if possible)
- 1 cup of chocolate chips

Instructions:

1. Preheat the oven to 350°F. Spread 2 large baking sheets with parchment paper.

2. In a large bowl, stir together the oats, seeds, almonds, and coconut. Add the vanilla, cinnamon, salt, and cocoa powder. Stir to combine.

3.Heat the maple syrup and coconut-oil in a low-heat frying pan. Pour the warm syrup and oil over the oat mixture and stir to coat. On the prepared baking sheets, spread the granola in even layers.

4. Bake for 15 to 18 minutes, scraping and mixing occasionally, then remove from the oven.

5. Put in the dried cherries and chocolate chips, then return to the oven, now turned off but still warm, and let the granola cool and dry completely.

Nutrition: Calories: 570 Total fat: 31g Cholesterol: 94mg Fiber: 2g Protein: 12g Sodium: 204mg

Creamy Raspberry Pomegranate Smoothie

Prep Time: 5 minutes

Cook Time: 5 minutes

Serve: 1

Ingredients:

- 1½ cups pomegranate juice
- ½ cup unsweetened coconut milk
- 1 scoop vanilla protein powder (plant-based if you need it to be dairy-free)
- 2 packed cups fresh baby spinach
- 1 cup frozen raspberries
- 1 frozen banana (see Tip)
- 1 to 2 tablespoons freshly compressed lemon juice

Instructions:

1. In a blender, combine the pomegranate juice and coconut milk. Add the protein powder and spinach. Give these a whirl to break down the spinach.

2. Add the raspberries, banana, and lemon juice, then top it off with ice. Blend until smooth and frothy.

Nutrition: Calories: 303 Total fat: 3g Cholesterol: 0mg Fiber: 2g
Protein: 15g Sodium: 165mg

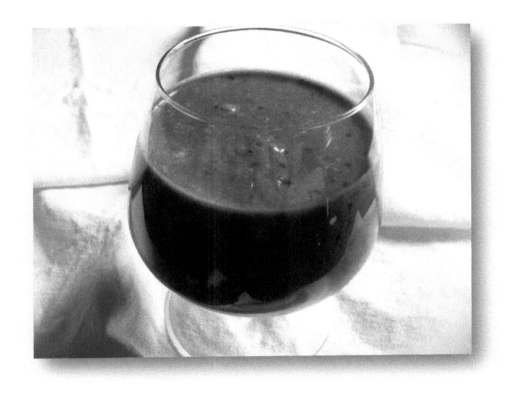

Mango Coconut Oatmeal

Prep Time: 5 minutes

Cook Time: 5 minutes

Serve: 2

Ingredients:

- 1½ cups water
- ½ cup 5-minute steel cut oats
- ¼ cup unsweetened canned coconut milk, plus more for serving (optional)
- 1 tablespoon pure maple syrup
- 1 teaspoon sesame seeds
- Dash ground cinnamon
- 1 mango, stripped, pitted, and divide into slices
- 1 tablespoon unsweetened coconut flakes

Instructions:

1. In a frying pan over high heat, boil water. Put the oats and lower the heat. Cook, occasionally stirring, for 5 minutes.

2. Put in the coconut milk, maple syrup, and salt to combine.

3. Get two bowls and sprinkle with the sesame seeds and cinnamon. Top with sliced mango and coconut flakes.

Nutrition: Calories: 373 Total fat: 11g Cholesterol: 0mg Fiber: 2g
Protein: 12g Sodium: 167mg

Spiced Sweet Potato Hash with Cilantro-Lime Cream

Prep Time: 20 minutes

Cook Time: 30 minutes

Serve: 2

Ingredients:

- For the cilantro-lime cream
- 1 avocado, halved and pitted
- ¼ cup packed fresh cilantro leaves and stems
- 2 tablespoons freshly squeezed lime juice
- 1 garlic clove, peeled
- 1 teaspoon kosher salt
- ½ teaspoon ground cumin
- 2 tablespoons extra-virgin olive oil
- For the hash
- ½ teaspoon kosher salt
- 1 large sweet potato, cut into ¾-inch pieces
- 2 tablespoons extra-virgin olive oil
- 1 onion, thinly sliced
- 2 garlic cloves, crushed
- 1 red bell pepper, thinly sliced
- 1 teaspoon ground cumin
- ¼ teaspoon ground turmeric
- Pinch freshly ground black pepper
- 2 tablespoons fresh cilantro leaves, chopped

- ½ jalapeño pepper, seeded and chopped (optional)
- Hot sauce, for serving (optional)

Instructions:

1. To make the cilantro-lime cream

2. Add the avocado flesh in a food compressor. Add the cilantro, lime juice, garlic, salt, and cumin. Whirl until smooth when the processor is running slowly, softly. Taste and adjust seasonings, as needed. If there is no food processor or blender for you,, simply mash the avocado well with a fork; the results will have more texture but will still work. Cover and refrigerate until ready to serve.

3. To make the hash

4. Boil saltwater in a medium pot over high heat. Add the sweet potato and cook for about 20 minutes until tender. Drain thoroughly.

5. Over low heat, heat the olive oil. In a large skillet until it shimmers. Add the onion and sauté for about 4 minutes until translucent. Put the garlic and cook, turning, for about 30 seconds. Add the cooked sweet potato and red bell pepper. Season the hash with cumin, salt, turmeric, and pepper. For 5 to 7 minutes, Saute until the sweet potatoes are golden and the red bell pepper is soft.

6. Divide the sweet potatoes between 2 bowls and spoon the sauce over them. Scatter the cilantro and jalapeño (if using) over each and serve with hot sauce (if using).

Nutrition: Calories: 520 Total fat: 43g Cholesterol: 0mg Fiber: 2g Protein: 12g Sodium: 1719mg

Open-Face Egg Sandwiches with Cilantro-Jalapeño spread

Prep Time: 20 minutes

Cook Time: 10 minutes

Serve: 2

Ingredients:

For the cilantro and jalapeño spread

- 1 cup filled up fresh cilantro leaves and stems (about 1 bunch)
- 1 jalapeño pepper, seeded and roughly chopped
- ½ cup extra-virgin olive oil
- ¼ cup pepitas (hulled pumpkin seeds), raw or roasted
- 2 garlic cloves, thinly sliced
- 1 tablespoon freshly squeezed lime juice
- 1 teaspoon kosher salt

For the eggs

- 4 large eggs
- ¼ cup milk
- ¼ to ½ teaspoon kosher salt
- 2 tablespoons butter

For the sandwich

- 2 slices bread
- 1 tablespoon butter

- 1 avocado, halved, pitted and divided into slices
  Microgreens or sprouts, for garnish

Instructions:

1. To make the cilantro and jalapeño spread

2. In a food processor, combine the cilantro, jalapeño, oil, pepitas, garlic, lime juice, and salt. Whirl until smooth. Refrigerate if making in advance; otherwise, set aside.

3. To make the eggs

4. In a medium bowl, whisk the eggs, milk, and salt.

5. Dissolve the butter in a skillet over low heat, swirling to coat the pan's bottom. Pour in the whisked eggs. Cook until they begin to set then, using a heatproof spatula, push them to the sides, allowing the uncooked portions to run into the bottom of the skillet. Continue until the eggs are set.

6. To assemble the sandwiches

7. Toast the bed and spread it with butter.

8. Spread a spoonful of the cilantro-jalapeño spread on each piece of toast. Top each with scrambled eggs.

9. Arrange avocado over each sandwich and garnish with microgreens.

Nutrition: Calories: 711 Total fat: 4g Cholesterol: 54mg Fiber: 12g Protein: 12g Sodium: 327mg

Scrambled Eggs with Soy Sauce and Broccoli Slaw

Prep Time: 5 minutes

Cook Time: 10 minutes

Serve: 2

Ingredients:

- 1 tablespoon peanut oil, divided
- 4 large eggs
- ½ to 1 tablespoon soy sauce, tamari, or Bragg's liquid aminos
- 1 tablespoon water
- 1 cup shredded broccoli slaw or another shredded vegetable
- Kosher salt
- Chopped fresh cilantro for serving
- Hot sauce, for serving.

Instructions:

1. In a medium nonstick skillet or cast-iron skillet over medium heat, heat 2 teaspoons of peanut oil, swirling to coat the skillet.

2. In a small bowl, whip the eggs, soy sauce, and water until smooth. Pour the eggs into the pan and let the bottom set. Using a wooden spoon, spread the eggs from one side to the other a couple

of times so the uncooked portions on top pool into the bottom. Cook until the eggs are set.

3. In a medium container, stir together the broccoli slaw, the remaining 1 teaspoon of peanut oil, and a salt touch. Divide the slaw between 2 plates.

4. Top with the eggs and scatter cilantro on each serving. Serve with hot sauce.

Nutrition: Calories: 222 Total fat: 4g Cholesterol: 374mg Fiber: 2g Protein: 12g Sodium: 737mg

Tasty Breakfast Donuts

Prep Time: 5 minutes

Cook Time: 5 minutes

Serve: 4

Ingredients:

- 43 grams' cream cheese
- 2 eggs
- 2 tablespoons almond flour
- 2 tablespoons erythritol
- 1 ½ tablespoons coconut flour
- ½ teaspoon baking powder
- ½ teaspoon vanilla extract
- 5 drops Stevia (liquid form)
- 2 strips bacon, fried until crispy

Instructions:

1. Rub coconut oil over the donut maker and turn it on.

2. Pulse all ingredients except bacon in a blender or food processor until smooth (should take around 1 minute).

3. pour batter into the donut maker, leaving 1/10 in each round for rising.

4. Leave for 3 minutes before flipping each donut. When you pierce them, leave for another 2 minutes or until the fork comes out clean.

5. Take donuts out and let cool.

6. Repeat steps 1-5 until all batter is used.

7. Crumble bacon into bits and use to top donuts.

Nutrition: Calories: 60 Fat: 5g Carbs: 1g Fiber: 0g Protein: 3g

Gluten -Free Pancakes

Prep Time: 5 minutes

Cook Time: 2 minutes

Serve: 2

Ingredients:

- 6 eggs
- 1 cup low-fat cream cheese
- 1 1/12; teaspoons baking powder
- 1 scoop protein powder
- 1/4; cup almond meal
- ¼ teaspoon salt

Instructions:

1. Combine dry ingredients in a food processor. Add the eggs one after another and then the cream cheese. Edit until you have a blast.

2. Lightly grease a skillet with spray and place over medium-high heat.

3. Pour the batter into the pan. Turn the pan gently to create round pancakes.

4. Cook for about 120 seconds on each side.

5. Serve pancakes with your favorite topping.

Nutrition: Dietary Fiber: 1g Net Carbs: 5g Protein: 25g Total Fat: 14g Calories: 288

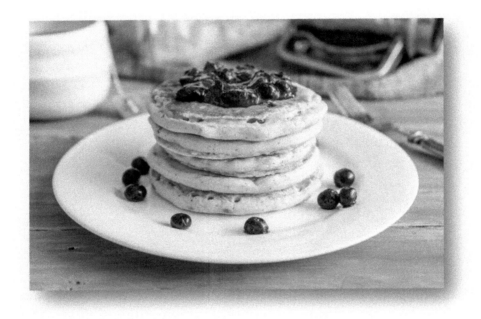

Mushroom & Spinach Omelet

Prep Time: 20 minutes

Cook Time: 20 minutes

Serve: 3

Ingredients:

- 2 tablespoons butter, divided
- 6-8 fresh mushrooms, sliced, 5 ounces
- Chives, chopped, optional
- Salt and pepper, to taste
- 1 handful baby spinach, about 1/2 ounce
- Pinch garlic powder
- 4 eggs, beaten
- 1-ounce shredded Swiss cheese,

Instructions:

1. In a very large saucepan, sauté the mushrooms in 1 tablespoon of butter until soft. Season with salt, pepper and garlic.

2. Remove the pan from the mushrooms and keep warm. Once the egg is almost out, place the cheese over the middle of the tortilla.

4. Fill the cheese with spinach leaves and hot mushrooms. Let cook for about a minute for the spinach to start to wilt. Fold the tortilla's empty side carefully over the filling and slide it onto a plate and sprinkle with chives, if desired.

5. Alternatively, you can make two tortillas using half the mushroom, spinach, and cheese filling in each.

Nutrition: Calories: 321 Fat: 26g Protein: 19g Carbohydrate: 4g Dietary Fiber: 1g

Gluten-Free Pancakes

Prep Time: 5 minutes

Cook Time: 2 minutes

Serve: 2

Ingredients:

- 6 eggs
- 1 cup low-fat cream cheese
- 1 1/12; teaspoons baking powder
- 1 scoop protein powder
- 1/4; cup almond meal
- ¼ teaspoon salt

Instructions:

1. Combine dry ingredients in a food processor. Add the eggs one after another and then the cream cheese. Edit until you have a blast.

2. Lightly grease a cooking spray skillet and position it over medium-high heat.

3. Pour the batter into the pan. Turn the pan gently to create round pancakes.

4. Cook on each side for about 2,5 minutes.

Nutrition: Dietary Fiber: 1g Net Carbs: 5g Protein: 25g Total Fat: 14g Calories: 288

Sweey and Smoked Salmon

Prep Time: 35 minutes

Cook Time: 1 hour

Serve: 8

Ingredients:

- 2 tablespoons light brown sugar
- 2 tablespoons smoked peppers
- 1 tablespoon shaved lemon peel
- Sare Kosar
- Freshly chopped black pepper Salmon fillets on the skin 1/2 kilogram

Instructions:

1. Soak a large plate (about 15 cm by 7 inches) in water for 1 to 2 hours.

2. It is heated over medium heat. Combine sugar, pepper, lemon zest, and 1/2 teaspoon of salt and pepper in a bowl. Mix the salmon with the salt and rub the mixture of spices in all parts of the meat.

3. Put the salmon on the wet plate, skin down — oven, covered, in the desired color, 25 to 28 minutes for medium.

Nutrition: Calories: 321 Total fat: 4g Cholesterol: 54mg Fiber: 2g Protein: 12g Sodium: 337mg

Vitamina C Smoothie Cubes

Prep Time: 5 minutes

Cook Time: 8 hours to chill

Serve: 1

Ingredients:

- 1/8 large papaya
- 1/8 mango
- 1/4 cups chopped pineapple, fresh or frozen
- 1/8 cup raw cauliflower florets, fresh or frozen
- 1/4 large navel oranges, peeled and halved
- 1/4 large orange bell pepper stemmed, seeded, and coarsely chopped

Instructions:

1. Halve the papaya and mango, remove the pits, and scoop their soft flesh into a high-speed blender.

2. Add the pineapple, cauliflower, oranges, and bell pepper. Blend until smooth.

3. Evenly divide the puree between 2 (16-compartment) ice cube trays and place them on a level surface in your freezer. Freeze for at least 8 hours.

4. The cubes can be left in the ice cube trays until use or transferred to a freezer bag. The frozen cubes are good for about

three weeks in a standard freezer or up to 6 months in a chest freezer.

Nutrition: Calories: 96, Fat: 1 g, Protein: 2 g, Carbohydrates: 24 g, Fiber: 4 g

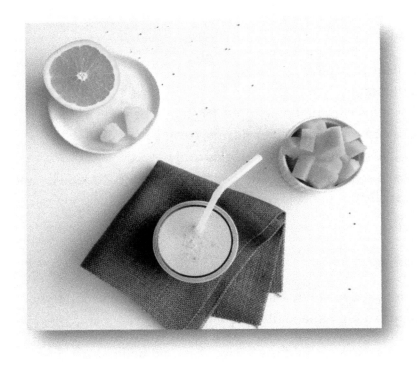

Polenta with Seared Pears

Prep Time: 10 minutes

Cook Time: 50 minutes

Serve: 1

Ingredients:

- One cup water, divided, plus more as needed
- 1/2 cups coarse cornmeal
- One tablespoon pure maple syrup
- 1/4 tablespoon molasses
- 1/4 teaspoon ground cinnamon
- 1/2 ripe pears, cored and diced
- 1/4 cup fresh cranberries
- 1/4 teaspoon chopped fresh rosemary leaves

Instructions:

1. In a pan, cook 5 cups of water to a simmer.

2. While whisking continuously to avoid clumping, slowly pour in the cornmeal. Cook, often stirring with a heavy spoon, for 30 minutes. The polenta should be thick and creamy.

3. While the polenta cooks, in a saucepan over medium heat, stir together the maple syrup, molasses, Whit the remaining 1/4 cup of water and when paired, the cinnamon. Bring it to a simmer. Add

the pears and cranberries. Cook for 10 minutes, occasionally stirring, until the pears are tender and start to brown.

4. Remove from the heat. Stir in the rosemary and let the mixture sit for 5 minutes. If it is too thick, add another 1/4 cup of water and return to the heat.

5. Top with the cranberry-pear mixture.

Nutrition: Calories: 282, Fat: 2 g, Protein: 4 g

Bell-Pepper Corn Wrapped in Tortilla

Prep Time: 5 minutes

Cook Time: 15 minutes

Serve: 1

Ingredients:

- 1/4 small red bell pepper, chopped
- 1/4 small yellow onion, diced
- 1/4 tablespoon water
- 1/2 cobs grilled corn kernels
- One large tortilla
- One-piece commercial vegan nuggets, chopped
- Mixed greens for garnish

Instructions:

1. Preheat the Instant Crisp Air Fryer to 400°F.

2. In a skillet heated over medium heat, sauté the vegan nuggets and the onions, bell peppers, and corn kernels. Set aside.

3. Place filling inside the corn tortillas.

4. Lock the air fryer lid. Fold the tortillas and place inside the Instant Crisp Air Fryer, cook for 15 minutes until the tortilla wraps are crispy.

5. Serve with mixed greens on top.

Nutrition: Calories: 548, Fat: 20.7g, Protein: 46g

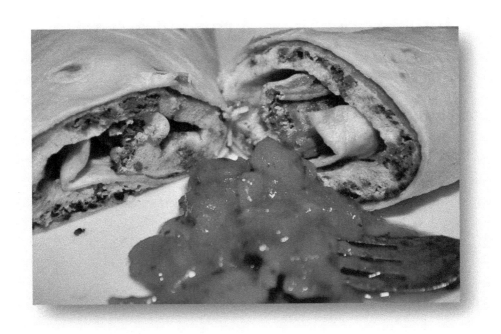

Eggplant Curry

Prep Time: 5 minutes

Cook Time: 30 minutes

Serve: 2

Ingredients:

- ½ tbsp. pepper
- ½ cups coconut milk (1 cup = 250ml)
- tin tomatoes (chopped) (roughly 14oz./400g)
- tbsp. Ground coriander
- tbsp. turmeric
- 1 tbsp. gram masala powder or curry powder
- clove garlic
- 1 red onion
- tbsp. Olive oil
- ½ tbsp. salt
- 1 aborigine (medium)
- Optional:
- tbsp. sugar (or 1-2 tbsp. mango chutney)

Instructions:

1.Cook as per packet directions when using rice.

2.Break your aubergine into tiny cubes. Fry with olive oil in a wide pan over high heat for 3-4 minutes. Mix well enough that it won't smoke.

3.Meanwhile, chop-the onion, and put it in as well. Put it back to medium heat and cook for 5-6 minutes.

4.Crush the garlic or dice it.

5.Garlic, curry powder, turmeric, and ground cilantro should be mixed in. Cook, stirring well, for the next 3-4 minutes.

6.Add in the sliced tomatoes and coconut milk. Add salt.

7.Boil for 15 minutes, roughly.

8.The coconut milk gets thicker, so when it is at the right consistency for you, stop cooking.

9.If you like it a little-sweeter, stir in the honey or mango chutney.

10. Serve according to taste, with salt and pepper.

Authentic Vegan Banana Pancakes

Prep Time: 5 minutes

Cook Time: 15 minutes

Serve: 4

Ingredients:

- 2 tbsp. Chia seeds
- ripe, med-sized banana
- tbsp. baking powder
- ⅓ cup wholemeal flour
- pinch salt
- cup soy milk (or your fave None-dairy)
- tbsp. olive oil (or coconut oil work great)
- cup rolled oats

Instructions:

1.Put all the products into a large bowl and use a hand blender to mix them.

2.In a None-stick pan, spray or drizzle with oil and scatter around with a paper towel. Heat (do not go higher!) at low-medium heat.

3.Place about a tiny volume of the batter. The pancakes should be tiny and fluffy.

4.Put a lid-on-it and let it softly steam the pancake. The other hand is through until the side facing you starts bubbling. Time for tossing! The smallest is a spatula.

5.Let the other side cook when turned, too. After a minute or two, take a look at the underside with the spatula. It is ready when it is good and brown (but not burnt!). Woo! Only repeat.

6.If you have a big pan, it's easy to simultaneously cook two or three small pancakes. Alternatively, if you experience a single flash, you should cook at the same time with two pans. Serve directly, or stack the pancakes in a warm oven on a tray before you're ready to eat.

African Peanut Soup

Prep Time: 15 minutes

Cook Time: 10 minutes

Serve: 3

Ingredients:

- cup brown rice (uncooked)
- A few dashes hot sauce
- tbsp. Soy sauce
- clove garlic
- small carrot
- tbsp. tomato paste
- handful of peanuts
- 3-4 tbsp. peanut butter
- ½ medium courgette (zucchini)
- ½ red onion
- cups vegetable broth
- 0.2 inches ginger, fresh (0.2 inches = 0.5 cm = ½ tbsp. powdered ginger)

Instructions:

1.Prepare the brown rice.

2.Put to the boil 700ml of vegetable broth.

3.Split the cabbage, carrot, and courgette and add them to the broth

4.Garlic and gingeer are also added to the broth.

5.Put in the peanuts.

6.Add some peanut butter and tomato paste to your mixture.

7.Add some soy sauce last but ensure it's not still too salty.

8.Let the rice boil until it is done.

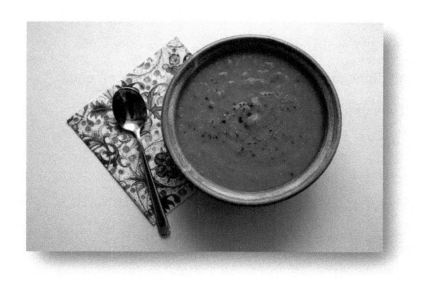

Zucchini Ravioli

Prep Time: 20 minutes

Cook Time: 25 minutes

Ingredients:

- 1 cup 257 grams of sauce with marinara
- 3 Medium zucchini, washed + dried with cut off ends
- 1 Tbsp of olive oil
- 2 cups 60 grams of fresh and washed spinach
- 2 Cloves 1 Tsp of chopped garlic
- 1 cup of 250 grams of whole ricotta milk
- 2 Tbsps of sliced fresh basil for garnishing
- 1 cup of cherry tomatoes 150 grams
- 1/2 cup of 56 grams of mozzarella (shredded into chunks)
- 2 Tsps 10 grams Parmesan grated

Instructions:

1. Oven preheat to 425 ° F.

2. On the bottom of a broad roasting dish, spread out the marinara sauce.

3. Use a mandolin or vegetable peeler to make your zucchini noodles. Peel the zucchini into strips 1/4 of an inch wide. Spread them out and sprinkle with salt on a surface lined with a paper towel. Set aside the remaining ingredients as you prepare.

4. Apply the olive oil to a medium-sized skillet and bring low heat to medium. Add the spinach, then cook until it is wilted. Add the garlic to the saucepan and cook until fragrant, to prevent burning, for a minute or two, stirring all the time. Switch off the fire, and remove the fire burner from the pan.

5. Along with the ricotta and chopped basil, add the spinach and garlic to a dish. Stir to blend.

6. Give your sliced zucchini back and blot away the excess moisture.

7. Take three zucchini strips at a time, and lay them on a clean surface. Layout the first two strips to form a 't' minus case. Line the top stripe of the zucchini with the lower sheet. Apply about 1 tbsp of the ricotta mixture to the zucchini core. To make little 'ravioli' packets, fold the ends of the strips over the ricotta mixture. Continue with the rest of the cheese/zucchini.

8. Switch the folded zucchini to the roasting plate and put the marinara/tomatoes on top. Along with the mozzarella & parmesan, scatter the tomatoes over the top.

9. 20 Minutes to bake in the oven. Broil and blister the tomatoes for an additional 2 minutes and then remove.

10. It is necessary to wait for it to cool down for 5 minutes before serving and enjoy! If required, sprinkle with extra basil.

Nutrition: calories: 193; cholesterol: 35mg; sodium: 422mg; carbohydrates: 10g; fiber: 2g; sugar: 6g; protein: 11g

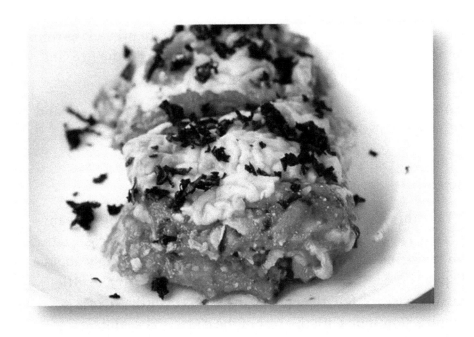

Lean & Green Tofu Stir-Fry

Prep Time: 10 min

Cook Time: 12 min

Ingredients:

- Olive oil for 2 tbsp
- 1/4 cup of White oignon
- 1/2 cup Oyster champignon (cutted into large pieces)
- 1/2 Green bell pepper (cutted into large pieces)
- 3 Rapini stalk, broccoli raab, raw (cutted into large pieces)
- 1/3 cup of Edamame frozen (soybeans)
- Tofu 227 gm, standard, extra firm (pressed and cutted into bite size cubes)
- 1 (minced)Garlic clove
- 3 tsp Yeast nutrition
- Oyster Sauce 1 tbsp
- 1 Tbsp Soja sauce with low sodium
- 5 Cherry Tomatoes
- 4 Cup Spinach for Infant
- Hot sauce 1 tsp

- 1/4 cup of (cut) Peanuts

Instructions:

1. Over medium pressure, spray a non-stick skillet with cooking spray and pressure.

2. Add the onion and mushrooms and saute for around 2-3 minutes until the onions are translucent and the mushrooms have softened.

3. For 3-4 minutes, add the green pepper, rapini, and edamame and sauté.

4. Connect the tofu and garlic to your skillet now. Toss to mix and cook for another 1-2 minutes.

5. Fill the pan with your oyster sauce, soy sauce, and nutritional yeast. Remove until well concealed.

6. Add the tomatoes and spinach. Cook for another 2-3 minutes before the spinach begins to wilt slightly.

7. Place sriracha and chopped peanuts on top. Enjoy!

Zucchini Lasagna

Prep Time: 40 mins

Cook Time: 30 mins

Ingredients*:*

For the zucchini layer:

- 5 Medium size zucchinis

- Cooking Spray With Olive Oil

- 1 1/2 tbsp kosher salt Diamond Crystal divided 1/2 tbsp split black pepper

- 1/2 tbsp powdered garlic

For the beef layer:

- Olive oil for 1 tbsp

- With 1 lb. Lean beef (85/15)

- 1 tbsp of garlic, minced

- 1 1/3 cup split marinara sauce

For the ricotta layer:

- 15 oz of room temperature whole milk ricotta cheese

- 2 large eggs

- 1/2 cup of chopped fresh basil

Topping:

- 8 oz of shredded part-skim split mozzarella cheese

Instructions:

Grill the zucchini slices:

1. Heat the grill and oven to 350 degrees F on medium heat. Long-slice the zucchinis into 1/4-inch-thick strips, get 6 slices out of each zucchini and discard the ends.

2. Spray olive oil on the zucchini slices and sprinkle with 1/2 tsp kosher salt, 1/8 tsp black-pepper, and 1/2 tsp garlic powder.

3. Grill the slices of zucchini, in lots, on each side for 2-3 minutes or until golden and firm, not browned and crisp. To soak up more humidity, spread them on clean kitchen towels.

Cook the beef:

1. In a large skillet over heat, heat the olive oil for about 2 minutes. Add the beef, minced garlic, kosher salt 1/2 tsp, and black pepper 1/4 tsp.

2. Cook, stirring to break up the beef with a spoon, until the meat is no longer raw, about five minutes. Return the meat to the pot and apply 1 cup of marinara sauce to the mixture, then drain in the colander. Turn off the flame and put yourself aside.

Prepare the ricotta layer:

1. In a medium bowl with a fork, combine the ricotta, eggs, basil, and the remaining kosher salt and black pepper together.

Assemble the lasagna:

1. Spread out the remaining 1/3 of a cup of marinara sauce on the bottom of a 9 X 13 baking dish. It is also possible to use a slightly smaller baking dish, such as a dish that measures 11 X 7 inches.

2. On top of the marinara sauce, add a layer of zucchini on top, then a third of the mixture of ricotta, a third of the mixture of meat, and a third of the shredded mozzarella cheese.

3. Repeat, in the opposite direction, arrange the zucchini slices: zucchini, 1/3 ricotta, 1/3 meat mixture, 1/3 mozzarella.

4. Add one extra layer of zucchini: zucchini, ricotta, meat mix, more zucchini, and mozzarella, and repeat for the last time.

Bake the lasagna:

1.Bake, uncovered, for about 31 minutes, until the cheese is golden. If desired and if your dish is broiler-safe, you can finish by broiling for 1-2 minutes on high to brown the cheese. For 10 minutes, Until serving, let stand.

Garlic Shrimp Zucchini Noodles

Prep Time: 15 mins

Cook Time: 15 mins

Ingredients:

- 2 Medium zucchini
- Shrimp shelled and de-veined 1 pound
- 2 Tbsp butter
- 3 sliced Garlic cloves
- Parmesan cheese: 3/4 cup
- Kosher salt or sea salt
- Black chili
- (1/4 tsp) red chili flakes
- lemon wedges

Instructions:

1. Using the vegetable spiraliser or julienne peeler to cut the zucchini into spirals or noodle strands. Put the noodles aside.

2. Over medium-high heat, heat a wide pan. Melt the olive oil/butter, then add the garlic and shrimp. Cook the shrimp until it is cooked. Don't let it burn the garlic.

3. Add the zucchini noodles, and cook for around 3-5 minutes until tender. Zucchini noodles are very easy to cook, so taste a strand as you cook and determine how firm or "al-dente" the zucchini you want. Don't overcook the zucchini noodles, or they're going to turn into mush.

4. Remove the pan from the fire, add parmesan cheese, squeeze some lemon juice and sprinkle with salt and pepper to taste generous. Serve warm, then add chili flakes.

Nutrition: Calories: 257kcal | Carbohydrates: 4g | Protein: 31g | Fat: 12g| Cholesterol:313mg | Sodium: 1241mg | Potassium: 372mg | Sugar: 2g | Calcium: 406mg |Iron: 2.9mg

Tofu with Peas

Prep time: 15 minutes

Cook time: 8 minutes

Serve: 4

Ingredients:

- 1¼ cups unsweetened coconut milk
- 2 tablespoons curry paste
- 14 ounces firm tofu, pressed, drained, and cubed
- 1 tablespoon olive oil
- ½ teaspoons garam masala powder
- ½ teaspoons ground cumin
- ¼ teaspoons cayenne pepper
- ¼ teaspoons ground turmeric
- 1½ cups frozen green peas, thawed
- Salt, as required

Instructions:

1. In a bowl, add coconut milk and curry paste and mix until smooth.

2. Add the oil in Instant Pot and select "Sauté". Then add the garam masala, cumin, cayenne and turmeric and cook for about 30 seconds.

3. Stir in tofu cubes and cook for about 2 minutes.

4. Press "Cancel" and stir in the coconut milk mixture, peas and salt.

5. Secure the lid and switch to the location of the "Seal".

6. Cook on "Manual" with "High Pressure" for about 5 minutes.

7. Press "Cancel" and carefully do a "Quick" release.

8. Remove the lid and serve hot.

Nutrition: Calories: 321 | fat: 24.8g | protein: 12.2g | carbs: 13g | net carbs: 9g | fiber: 4g

Cheesy Spicy Bacon Bowls

Prep Time: 10 minutes

Cook Time: 22 minutes

Serve: 12

Ingredients:

- 6 strips Bacon, pan-fried until cooked but still malleable
- 4 eggs
- 60 grams' cheddar cheese
- 40 grams' cream cheese, grated
- 2 Jalapenos, sliced and seeds removed
- 2 tablespoons coconut oil
- ¼ teaspoon onion powder
- ¼ teaspoon garlic powder
- Dash of salt and pepper

Instructions:

1. Preheat oven to 375 degrees Fahrenheit

2. In a bowl, beat together eggs, cream cheese, jalapenos (minus 6 slices), coconut oil, onion powder, garlic powder, and salt and pepper.

3. Using leftover bacon grease on a muffin tray, rubbing it into each insert. Place bacon-wrapped inside the parameters of each insert.

4. Pour the beaten mixture halfway up each bacon bowl.

5. Garnish each bacon bowl with cheese and leftover jalapeno slices (placing one on top of each).

6. Leave in the oven for about 22 minutes, or until the egg is thoroughly cooked and cheese is bubbly.

7. Remove from oven and let cool until edible.

Nutrition: Calories: 259 Fat: 24g Carbs: 1g Fiber: 0g Protein: 10g

Goat Cheese Zucchini Kale Quiche

Prep Time: 35 minutes

Cook Time: 1 hour 10 minutes

Serve: 4

Ingredients:

- 4 large eggs
- 8 ounces' fresh zucchini, sliced
- 10 ounces' kale
- 3 garlic cloves (minced)
- 1 cup of soy milk
- 1 ounce's goat cheese
- 1cup grated parmesan
- 1cup shredded cheddar cheese
- 2 teaspoons olive oil
- Salt & pepper, to taste

Instructions:

1. Preheat oven to 350°F.

2. Heat 1 TSP of olive-oil in a casserole dish over medium-high heat.

6. Slightly grease a baking dish with cooking spray and spread the kale leaves across the bottom. Add the zucchini and top with goat cheese.

7. Pour the egg, milk and parmesan mixture evenly over the other ingredients. Top with cheddar cheese.

8. Bake for 50–60 minutes until golden brown. Check the center of the quiche; it should have a solid consistency.

9. Let chill for a few minutes before serving.

Nutrition: Total Carbohydrates: 15g Dietary Fiber: 2g Net Carbs: 13g Protein: 19g Total Fat: 18g Calories: 290

Cream Cheese Egg Breakfast

Prep Time: 5 minutes

Cook Time: 5 minutes

Serve: 4

Ingredients:

- 2 eggs, beaten
- 1 tablespoon butter
- 2 tablespoons soft cream cheese with chives

Instructions:

1. Melt the butter in a small skillet. Add the eggs and cream cheese. Stir and cook to desired doneness.

Nutrition: Calories: 341 Fat: 31g Protein: 15g Carbohydrate: 0g Dietary Fiber: 3g

Avocado Red Peppers Roasted Scrambled Eggs

Prep Time: 10 minutes

Cook Time: 12 minutes

Serve: 3

Ingredients:

- 1/2 tablespoon butter
- Eggs, 2
- 1/2 roasted red pepper, about 1 1/2 ounces
- 1/2 small avocado, coarsely chopped, about 2 1/4 ounces
  Salt, to taste

Instructions:

1. Heat the butter over heat in a nonstick skillet. Break the eggs into the pan and break the yolks with a spoon. Sprinkle with a little salt.

2. Stir to stir and continue stirring until the eggs start to come out. Quickly add the bell peppers and avocado.

3. Cook and stir until the eggs suit your taste. Adjust the seasoning, if necessary.

Nutrition: Calories: 317 Fat: 26g Protein: 14g Dietary Fiber: 5g Net Carbs: 4g

Mushroom Quickie Scramble

Prep Time: 10 minutes

Cook Time: 10 minutes

Serve: 4

Ingredients:

- 3 small-sized eggs, whisked
- 4 pcs. bella mushrooms
- ½ cup of spinach
- ¼ cup of red bell peppers
- 2 deli ham slices
- 1 tablespoon of ghee or coconut oil
- Salt & pepper to taste

Instructions:

1. Chop the ham and veggies.

2. Put half a tbsp of butter in a frying pan and heat until melted.

3. Sauté the ham and vegetables in a frying pan, then set aside.

4. Get a new frying pan and heat the remaining butter.

5. Add the whisked eggs into the second pan while stirring continuously to avoid overcooking.

6. When the eggs are done, sprinkle with salt & pepper to taste.

7. Add the ham and veggies to the pan with the eggs.

8. Mix well.

9. Remove it from the burner and transfer it to a tray.

Nutrition: Calories: 350 Total Fat: 29 g Protein: 21 g Total Carbs: 5 g

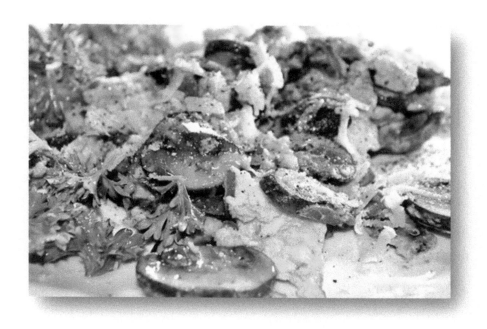

Coconut Coffee and Ghee

Prep Time: 10 minutes

Cook Time: 10 minutes

Serve: 5

Ingredients:

- ½ Tbsp. of coconut oil
- ½ Tbsp. of ghee
- 1 to 2 cups of preferred coffee (or rooibos or black tea, if preferred)
- 1 Tbsp. of coconut or almond milk

Instructions:

1. Place the almond (or coconut) milk, coconut oil, ghee and coffee in a blender (or milk frother).

2. mix for around 10 seconds or until the coffee turns creamy and foamy.

3. Pour contents into a coffee cup.

Nutrition: Calories: 150 Total Fat: 15 g Protein: 0 g Total Carbs: 0 g Net Carbs: 0 g

Yummy Veggie Waffles

Prep Time: 10 minutes

Cook Time: 9 minutes

Serve: 3

Ingredients:

- 3 cups raw cauliflower, grated
- 1 cup cheddar cheese
- 1 cup mozzarella cheese
- ½ cup parmesan
- 1/3 cup chives, finely sliced
- 6 eggs
- 1 teaspoon garlic powder
- 1 teaspoon onion powder
- ½ teaspoon chili flakes
- Dash of salt and pepper

Instructions:

1. Turn the waffle maker on.

2. Mix all the ingredients in a bowl.

3. Once the waffle maker is hot, distribute the waffle mixture into the insert.

4. Let cook for about 9 minutes, flipping at 6 minutes.

5. Remove from waffle maker and set aside.

6. Repeat the steps with the batter until it's gone (4 waffles should come out)

Nutrition: Calories: 390 Fat: 28g Carbs: 6g Fiber: 2g Protein: 30g

Omega 3 Breakfast Shake

Prep Time: 5 minutes

Cook Time: 5 minutes

Serve: 2

Ingredients:

- 1 cup vanilla almond milk (unsweetened)
- 2 tablespoons blueberries
- 1 ½ tablespoons flaxseed meal
- 1 tablespoon MCT Oil
- ¾ tablespoon banana extract
- ½ tablespoon chia seeds
- 5 drops Stevia (liquid form)
- 1/8 tablespoon Xanthan gum

Instructions:

1. In a blender, pulse vanilla almond milk, banana extract, Stevia, and 3 ice cubes.

2. When smooth, add blueberries and pulse.

3. Once blueberries are thoroughly incorporated, add flaxseed meal and chia seeds.

4. Let sit for 5 minutes.

5. After 5 minutes, pulse again until all ingredients are nicely distributed.

Nutrition: Calories: 264 Fats: 25g Carbs: 7g Protein: 4g

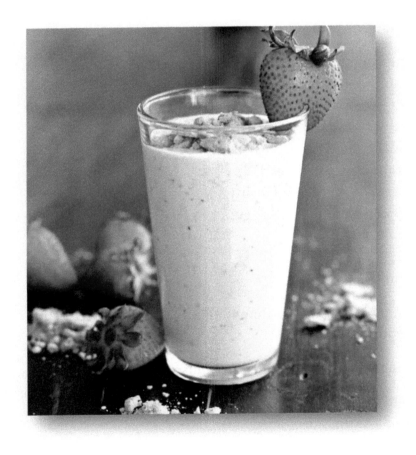

Bacon Spaghetti Squash Carbonara

Prep Time: 20 minutes

Cook Time: 40 minutes

Serve: 4

Ingredients:

- 1 small spaghetti squash
- 6 ounces' bacon (roughly chopped)
- 1 large tomato (sliced)
- 2 chives (chopped)
- 1 garlic clove (minced)
- 6 ounces' low-fat cottage cheese
- 1 cup Gouda cheese (grated)
- 2 tablespoons olive oil
- Salt and pepper, to taste

Instructions:

1. Preheat the oven to 350°F.

2. Cut the squash spaghetti in half, brush with some olive oil and bake for 20–30 minutes, skin side up. Remove from the oven and remove the core with a fork, creating the spaghetti.

3. In a pan, heat one tablespoon of olive oil. Cook the bacon for about 1 minute until crispy.

4. Quickly wipe out the pan with paper towels.

5. Heat another tablespoon of oil and sauté the garlic, tomato and chives for 2–3 minutes. Add the spaghetti and sauté for another 5 minutes, occasionally stirring to keep from burning.

6. Begin to add the cottage cheese, about 2 tablespoons at a time. If the sauce becomes thick, add about a cup of water. It should be smooth with the sauce but not too runny or thick. Allow cooking for another 3 minutes.

Nutrition: Calories: 305 Total Fat: 21g Net Carbs: 8g Protein: 18g

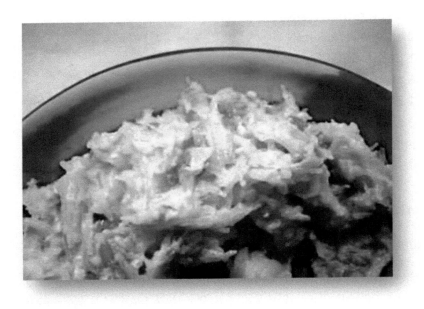

Lime Bacon Thyme Muffins

Prep Time: 10 minutes

Cook Time: 20 minutes

Serve: 3

Ingredients:

- 3 cups of almond flour
- 4 medium-sized eggs
- 1 cup of bacon bits
- 2 tsp. of lemon thyme
- ½ cup of melted ghee
- 1 tsp. of baking soda
- ½ tsp. of salt, to taste

Instructions:

1. Pre-heat oven to 350° F.

2. Put ghee in the mixing bowl and melt.

3. Add baking soda and almond flour.

4. Put the eggs in.

5. Add the lemon thyme (if preferred, other herbs or spices may be used).

6. Drizzle with salt.

7. Mix all ingredients well.

8. Sprinkle with bacon bits

9. Line the muffin pan with liners.

10. Spoon mixture into the pan, filling the pan to about ¾ full.

11. Bake for about 20 minutes. Test by inserting a toothpick into a muffin. If it comes out clean, then the muffins are done.

Nutrition: Calories: 300 Total Fat: 28 g Protein: 11 g Total Carbs: 6 g Fiber: 3 g

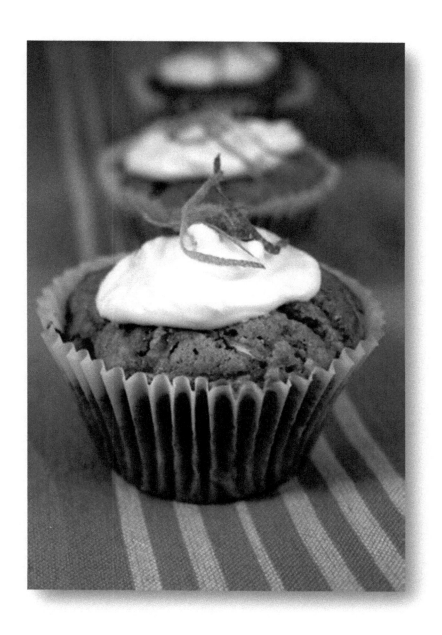

Lightning Source UK Ltd.
Milton Keynes UK
UKHW020706130521
383649UK00005B/74